Core Exercises for Men and Women

How to develop a ripped and functional core to release pain and boost strength

Konrad Obidoski

© Copyright 2015 by Konrad Obidoski - All rights reserved.

This document is geared towards providing exact and reliable information in regards to the topic and issue covered. The publication is sold with the idea that the publisher is not required to render accounting, officially permitted, or otherwise, qualified services. If advice is necessary, legal or professional, a practiced individual in the profession should be ordered.

- From a Declaration of Principles which was accepted and approved equally by a Committee of the American Bar Association and a Committee of Publishers and Associations.

reparation, damages, or monetary loss due to the information herein, either directly or indirectly.

Respective authors own all copyrights not held by the publisher.

The information herein is offered for informational purposes solely, and is universal as so. The presentation of the information is without contract or any type of guarantee assurance.

The trademarks that are used are without any consent, and the publication of the trademark is without permission or backing by the trademark owner. All trademarks and brands within this book are for clarifying purposes only and are the owned by the owners themselves, not affiliated with this document.

Table of Contents

Introduction

I want to thank you and congratulate you for Purchasing the book, *"Core exercises for men and women"*!

In the modern world everybody wants a washboard abs. Every person who exercises at least casually, from time to time, usually for two weeks after New Year's Eve and two weeks before summer pursues the goal of ripped stomach. Why then, if everybody is so health-conscious, the staggeringly high rate of injuries, bulged discs and snapped back? The term "snap city" was coined and functions on a daily basis in the Internet fitness community and there is a reason for that.

Most people today can't use their own body in a proper manner. This isn't surprising as it doesn't come with user's manual and the way we behave is mostly dictated by a world that requires "human resources" and not really humans themselves. I rarely meet people who have correct abdominal wall function. Back pain is the fastest spreading disease in the western world and statistically about 1 person out of 300 who suffers from it has an adequately functioning core.

The most prevalent reason is the inability to properly stabilize the core and recruit the muscles when needed, which often times has its source in improper training or faulty lifestyle. Not only this may cause decrease of athletic performance as the core is the central unit through which all forces are transferred, it can be the reason of severe and chronic pain that debilitates people's ability to experience life! So, whether you want to become a stronger athlete or be able to live painlessly, read on...

In this book we will break some common myth about core training, then briefly cover the functional anatomy of the core next outline the proper training techniques and go over to a progressive sequence of exercises to facilitate your healing or athletic development.

This book's aim is to provide a comprehensive guide to using and training your core as a functional unit. Every person should have and understanding of this topic as it may dictate the quality of your everyday life. However, athletes may benefit the most as this may help them to increase their results in the gym and protect them from injuries and prevent their sports life from crashing to a sudden halt.Thanks again for downloading this book, I hope you enjoy it!

Konrad Obidoski

Chapter 1
Core Conditioning and Training

Before going on to further things, let's talk about what is Core conditioning/training/sculpting. This is actually related to body shape building or enhancement; core training exercises are non-aerobic, and focused on muscle toning. Most of these exercises include strength and weight training along with the use of tool such as dumbbells and barbells and other gadgets.

Basically core conditioning is about making your body look good. In recent times, many men and women have jumped on this bandwagon with the aim of getting their muscles toned and look appealing. I am sure that many of you have looked at models in commercials or in print ads and hoped for abs or a toned stomach like they do.

Well, looking like a model requires a lot of time and energy and if you are willing to invest that, then it is no problem. However for people just looking for exercises build their core area and muscles, then this book might be of help. Core training focuses on the trunk muscles of the body, and developing those can be very effective for the overall workout routine as well. Having a strong core prevents injuries as well.

Core training not only builds the body shape but it is also good for maintaining bone density and posture. The good thing about these exercises is that anyone can do this if they are focused enough. All you need to do is set a target, if you want to build six-pack abs, then focus on doing the exercises that can help in that.

If you have ever tried some kind of a physical therapy, then you might already be familiar with the idea of strengthening the core. That is exactly what core conditioning is about. The muscles that lie at the core should be strong enough; these are the muscles in the abdominal area, lower back and pelvis, mainly those that lie between the rib cage and hips. The strength of these muscles is not just important for athletes and sportsmen, it is also important in daily life functioning.

Basic studies that began on the importance of working the core muscles began around in 1990s. They showed that people with healthy backs, when moving an arm or leg, were automatically contracting their core muscles. Based on the conclusions from those studies, experts stated that a well-coordinated and stable core are could not only stabilize the spine but also help give a firm base and support to all muscles movements in the body.

The core conditioning exercises are usually included in the overall fitness routine. They usually include twenty to thirty minute intensity workout and strength training sometimes only two or three times a week. This is relatively easy for novices and beginners, as they do not have to push themselves that hard.

To avoid injury and doing these training exercises the right way, one must make sure that the core strengthening exercises are done properly. The muscles should be aligned and progression from one workout routine to another should be maintained and adjusted according every individual's fitness and body type.

Consult a physical coach and gym instructor to supervise and help you through the exercises. And if you are a beginner working on starting the core training exercises, it is vital that you get yourself checked by a doctor before embarking on such a mission.

Some of the very basic exercises regarding core strengthening begin with the 'drawing in' of the body. Drawing in is basically a lying, sitting or standing position where the abdominal muscles are tightened by moving the navel area in towards the small of your back. The tailbone should also be tucked in slightly. Many instructors identify this part of the core training as 'bracing yourself', like prepare to get hit or take a punch.

This is drawing in position should only be attempted at least for ten to fifteen seconds before going on to do some core training.

Some of these very simple exercises include:

-The Basic Crunch

Just lie back, bend your knees and put your feet flat against the floor. Your fingertips should be placed at the top of your head. Tighten the abdominal muscles, and then take a curling position upwards. Lift the shoulder blades off the floor. Hold in that position for about ten to twenty seconds. Lower down halfway slowly, and then repeat. It is advised that you do fifteen to twenty basic crunches daily.

-The Plank

Lie on a mat, stomach down with the forearms resting. Draw in and tighten the abdominal muscles, then press up. Ensure that you can balance on the toes and elbows. Do not let the hips stick up or sag; the body should be positioned in a straight line from the head to the heels. Hold that position for about thirty seconds, then lower yourself and repeat for a couple more times. Try to increase the holding time till up to sixty seconds.

-The Bicycle

Lie on the floor, flat on the back. Place the fingertips at the back of the head and then tighten the abdominal muscles. In doing so, bring the knees up to almost a forty-five degree angle and then lift the shoulder blades off the floor. Turn the upper body to the left side, bring the right elbow towards the left knee and then extend the right leg. Switch the sides and bring the left elbow towards right knee. Continue the pedaling and take the total repetitions to sixteen or twenty. Try resting in between and then repeating. Make sure that you don't injure your neck or pull it.

Try using stability balls during exercise, the core muscles can perform greater due to it being unstable. And it is good for some exercises and better than a flat surface.

The leg and arm raise on such a ball is one such exercise that is very efficient for enhancing core muscle activity.

Lie on top of the ball so that the hips are over it and straighten your legs. The toes and fingers should be able to reach the floor comfortably. Tighten the abdominal muscles and then lift the right arm and left leg. Hold that position for five seconds, then rest. Repeat with the other side, that is the left arm and the right leg. Repeat till about eight to twelve times. If you want to do more, then try and lift the same leg and arm.

Konrad Obidoski

Core conditioning is the best way to look good without putting in too much time and energy into products or strenuous exercises. It makes you look healthy, in shape and yes even attain those much coveted six pack abs.

Chapter 2

Core Exercises for Beginners

If you are a beginner and looking to start on building your core area, here's what to know. If you are not that much familiar with core training, well it just about exercising all those areas that are not the arms and legs. This means that while working on your core, you will be focusing on areas that are; the abdomen, the glutes, pelvic muscles, inner abdominal muscles and the scapula.

The core is basically the area where the power is generated and flows in the body.

First try to understand what it is and what it does. As you know by now that it involves all the deep and intricate muscles of the abdominal and pelvic areas. The core acts as a center of force transfer, rather than the prime mover. It is like a stabilizer as well. People focus on training this part of a body as a prime mover; they do exercises like crunches rather than lifts, squats or pushups. By ignoring those aspects of muscles, the people miss out on more efficiency in movement, better health and strength gaining.

The core area must be looked as the part of the body that is responsible for producing force and controlling the ability to produce force. An expert has described core stability as possessing five components; strength, flexibility, endurance, motor control and function. Even if you miss out on working upon even one or two of these components, the entire workout becomes useless.

For example, if you take out motor control and function, the other components will be utterly useless, no matter how much focus you put in strength training or building up endurance.

It is important to focus on achieving core stability so that you can protect your spine, and avoid injury. Then it is advisable to move on to dynamic movements. It is also important to efficiently and effectively manage and produce the force during these dynamic movements. This is done through exercises like running, lifting Olympic weights or picking up heavy weights while keeping the back in a safe position.

Research has produced evidence that athletes, who have a higher stability of core, run a low risk of injury.

How to test the core stability is one question that would come to the mind of the readers. Well there are a few tests for that. There is the Functional Movement Screen, which produces results that are most effective.

-The Trunk Stability Push-Up Test

This test can be conducted as a simple fail or pass test.

First, to begin, go into a prone pushup position. The toes should be tucked in and you should be lying flat on the ground. The men who are attempting this particular should have the palm of their hands in line with their chin, while the women who take the test should place the palms in line with their collar bone or clavicle as it is called.

Now keep in mind that you should do this in a single motion; a pushup while keeping the body straight. The hands should be shoulder width apart. You can use a rod or a pipe just for evaluation, to assess the body shape and core area.

The passing criteria for this test is; if the person is able to maintain a proper start position, as in the hands do not slide down or lower. The chest and stomach leave the ground at the same time. The spinal alignment has been maintained as the body moved as a single unit; this is where the rod or pipe can be used to see if it is proper.

If the individual does not meet the criteria then the test is seen as failing. You can have a maximum of three tries ad if one can pass this during those then they can move on to the strength determining tests.

It is important to have good core stability as it helps with the progression of the rest of the movements.

The core strength tests are more of exercises like the plank and side plank.

-The plank and side planks are good evaluators of the core strength, while the knees to chests and toes.

As you have read the plank is fairly basic and easy to do. However, when you are doing it for testing, try holding the position for ninety seconds. Maintain a strict posture, flat back and level the hips. Use a dowel if you can to assess posture alignment.

If you are unable to or struggling to maintain proper alignment then try doing this; try assuming the prone position, with the elbows located under the shoulders. Flex the quads, raise the knees off the floor, press the buttocks tightly, retract and tighten the abs as well.

When all of this done correctly, you will be able to lock the hips ensuring a flat back and lower area.

The side planks are also an effective way of strength testing. Hold the position for sixty seconds. In doing a side planks, place the elbow directly under the shoulder, while both feet must be stacked on top of each other. The spinal alignment must be straight, whether maintained vertically or horizontally.

-The knees to chest and toes to bar exercises are the best way to find out how strong the core is. Complete five strict knees to chest successfully if you want to pass this test or go for five toes to bar if you want to gain a substantial scoring.

If you are hanging from a pull up bar, ensure that your shoulders are aligned properly or you will risk injury otherwise. The slowly lift the toes towards the bar. Then slowly bring them down with control and without swinging.

You can do something similar with knees to the chest routine. Instead of toes you can try and bring up your knees.

Repeat this five times at least.

If you want to pass this test, it is essential that you remain completely in control of the movements, do not increase momentum or speed of motion while doing the exercise, and also remain without any pain.

You can also do deadlifts. Ask your gym instructor or supervisor for the weight chart and life according to that. The chart will have weights according to the body weight of an individual and their level of gym fitness. For example, a person who is untrained or a novice will have more weights to life than someone who is trained or at a further level of fitness.

A common mistake that novices make is that they get attracted by the dazzle, that is the building of abs. Due to this their training can be ineffective and pretty much not of any use if it does not involve the working of other muscles. Basic core exercises like the plank or crunches are attempted to get those abs that can become the envy of many. But that is just doing core training for all the wrong reasons and is quite a terrible method of attempting this.

Crunches and sit ups when done very vigorously can not only be ineffective in building the core, but also be very dangerous for the spinal cord and just the spine in general. Crunches also don't work like that, contrary to the popular opinion. The abdomen muscles work in a different way then what people think. Their main function is to support the spine, and basically preventing it from spinning, twisting and flexing to the other side.

To train the core and in an effective way, it is essential the one understands the basics. Start slowly and steadily build up a foundation. All the muscles need to work together, think of it like a team or setting up a base for your house. The structure should be concrete, provide safety and be solid. Similarly, so should be the core area.

Do not rush and miss out on any step, and begin with charting out a simple plan first. You are probably familiar with planks and other basic exercises that have been mentioned above.

Those are the well-known ones, the ones that I will talk about here are those that are little known but can go a long way in strengthening and building the core muscles.

-The first one is Tummy Vacuums.

These are simple and effective core powering exercises. They are especially good for beginners/novices, women who have had a couple of children and people who really have not been that active in exercising since long.

Tummy vacuums help in the reconditioning the transverse abdominal muscles so that they can brace and support the spine during movement. These muscles are basically like a belt with weight that has to be engaged when a person attempts to life something or move. If you are inactive or have been through pregnancy then chances are that the transverse muscles are not functioning or have very little function left in them.

For people who sit for long or are 'couch potatoes', their transverse abdominal muscles become dormant and with time forget how to engage in movement or activity.

Getting these muscles to function properly again is a must. Think of it like oiling a car engine. To get these to work well again, these tummy vacuums can do wonders.

-The Clam Shells

The strongest muscles within the body are the glutes, those are the butt muscles. If they are functioning and working properly, they can go a long way in stabilizing and driving the power in movement, especially when it comes to athletics.

But when they are not working well, they can cause weakness, pain and muscular imbalance in the body.

Most beginners who start core training do have glutes that work to the fullest. It can differ individually, for some people their glutes might function properly for others they might not function at all. When the latter is happening, the hip flexors start taking over, hamstrings get tight, and there is a lot of pressure that can be put on the lower back. This can make other lower body exercises also very difficult. Glutes become weakened further, and require a lot of time to get better.

The Clam shells are an important exercise as far as glutes are concerned. They can go a long way in getting the glutes to function again. They are quite simple to do as well so the beginners will have little problem in attempting these.

-Dead Bugs

The name sounds interesting. The exercise is as well.

It is a very effective trunk stabilizing and core building exercise. Not only does it help with the core conditioning, it is excellent for building up stability in the trunk and hips as well.

Dead bugs can help in preparing people and getting them readied for crawling exercises too. They are helpful in building the coordination in the cross crawling exercises, since they are essentially mimicking the leg and hand movements. These are only performed on the back rather than the hand and feet.

-The Band Anti-Rotation

The abdominal muscles have three essential functions; anti-rotation, anti-lateral flexion and anti-extension.

The mistake most people make is that they leave out anti-rotation exercises. Most of them will include routines that will work upon the anti-lateral flexion and anti-extension, but they will overlook the rotation.

This is why you can try the anti-rotations resistance bands. They are effective and simple, can be done at home and as well as the gym. If you do not have a resistance band or want to try something different, try using a cable machine.

-Bird Dog

This is a very good and interesting exercise. It is excellent for core stability as it utilizes a number of functions at once. It works on both the anti-rotation and anti-extension, improving of coordination and movements, and also works up both the glutes and shoulders muscles.

Like the dead bug, this is an exercise that can be of help in the cross crawling exercises.

This is a great exercise and can be very beneficial for you.

Now that you know about all these exercises and are wondering where to start, here's what you can do.

Easy and simple to follow, stick to this and you will be able to see the effects yourself within a very short time.

Attempt to do each and every one of those exercises in this routine; Bird Dog is one position that can be held for ten seconds, and for eight repetitions. Band anti-rotation can also be done for the same eight repetitions with ten seconds hold. Do the dead bugs for eight repetitions for each side, alternating each rep with sides. Clamshells can be done for ten reps per each side and each should be of a ten second hold. Do the Tummy vacuums for five second holds and eight reps.

When you are performing these exercises as a routine turn, rest for one minute in between every cycle. Try doing up to three cycles and repeating each exercise for a couple of times.

If you are doing these as a warm up, then just reduce the cycles for up to two but one will be fine as well.

Training the core area is not a difficult task and if you do these exercises and follow routines as instructed then you will see how easy it becomes.

Konrad Obidoski

Chapter 3

Actually Strengthening the Core

Core strengthening is not just about crunching, leg raises and weight lifting. There is one very important aspect of this, core stabilizing exercise. The core stability is integral to the functioning of the core.

Now for people who have read so far are aware of the basics of core functioning. The core has many more muscles and not just the four that are commonly associated with it. Usually people building up on core strength focus on the muscles in the abdominal, these are the rectus abdominis, internal or external oblique and transverse abdominis, the mutlifidis and erector spinae. These are just some that are worked upon the most, there are others also like hip flexors and glute muscles.

The core is very closely related to spinal movement, and its stability can be judged by the rotation of the spine. It is said that if the spine is moving, the core is strengthening, and not stabilizing. And any of the muscle involved in keeping the spine stable is a core muscle.

Suppose for example, if you hold a weight in your right hand, your body will start to dip towards the right. There will be an opposing force produced that will try to balance the body and prevent it from dipping towards the left. This force will be produced from the legs and lower abdominal area of the body. If you are able to retain yourself in balance and the spine remains erect then the core is stable.

To being able to retain the spine is called core stability.

All those muscles that were involved in keeping the spine neutral are core muscles. And when it comes to strengthening them, there are some very particular exercises advised.

Some of the experts think that rolling and crawling are great core stability exercises. They have noticed that indulging in such exercises have brought about very positive effects on people.

So why is so much importance given to something so basic as crawling?

Well it is one exercise that is the basis for all athletic activities further on. Observer that when you crawl, your arms and legs move in the opposition with each other. In the prone crawling position, you are able to feel the working of the muscles used in stabilizing the spine even more than usual, since there is the extra pressure of the gravity working upon them.

An exercise like the plank is very good for this purpose too. It helps stabilize the core and it is primarily about abdominal stability. This is a good way but too easy, in order to really stabilize the core, you might need to up the ante. Try doing the plank with an arm or a leg raised to test further stability.

If you get good with these, then move on to the other crawling exercises. They are low intensity and low speed exercises that actually allow a person to feel how their body is performing. They also enable a person to attain better movement and coordination within their exercise routine.

Like the hips should stay absolutely flat and in position, without rocking from one side to another or swinging. Knees should be coming out in straight and forward position while the spine should be able to stay flat throughout each exercise.

There are many types of crawling activities that you can indulge in, but after doing the easy ones, try to progress onto the further hard ones.

To challenge the body do this one single exercise. It involves using one heavy kettlebell weight and doing the dipping experiment. Try to make sure that the spine remains completely neutral during this. The reason why a single heavy weight has been advised is because that's what is going to pull the spine and force a dipping position. Your task is to stop that from happening.

Do this for core stabilizing once you are able to do the easy movements smoothly.

If you do not understand how this works then let me explain it to you.

Take a goblet squat, think about all the muscles that are involved in that exercise and what happens to the core stability when one attempts to this. The abdominal muscles work towards preventing the person from having a spine lumbar flexion, that is the upper body goes into a drooping position. Now during this the back muscles in keeping the spine up and straight. The thigh muscles also have their own work to do in keeping the abdominal and spine from going into the flexion and droop down. Even the muscles in the feet are working towards providing a good arching position.

Now take the kettlebell weight. Those are exactly the muscles that work when a person is holding this weight. You have to use all those muscle and counter the lumbar spinal flexion. The side that carries the weight has to counter the extra force that comes with the use of the weight.

A person can work even harder on this by trying some exercises like quick lift. The one hand swing is one of those. Compared to exercises like the plank, the one hand swing can put the body through some intense training. The opposite side to the weight can experience a lot of voluntary muscle contraction. When these two opposing forces are produced, the body tries to remain stable and as balanced as possible. A lot of effort goes into stabilizing the spine. Through this exercise the body learns how stabilize the spine and core area quickly and with each progression.

The swing does not even require that much of a heavy weight, use something and even that can generate the required forces in a core stabilizing exercise.

These are some of the core stabilizing exercises; a stable core means a strong one as well.

For people looking to move on further, here are some core strengthening exercises that can be done as well. They might be a bit out of the box but in this chapter that's what we have been focusing on. Something different, yet easily done and effective we have also talked about pushing yourself and trying new things. So here are some exercises that you can try; isometric holds, crawling, single sided exercises and levers, and throwing.

-The Isometric holds

By now you know everything that is to know about a plank, here's another interesting piece of information. It is also one of the most commonly known isometric exercises involving the core. It is essential that you learn the plank movement properly and do it effectively. It is one of the first and foremost exercises taught at gyms and usually incorporated in the entire workout routines.

Try to mix up ways to do the plank and hopefully you will not get bored of doing it over and over again.

-Movement of Crawling

You have already learnt important crawling is as an activity to stabilize the core. If you have tried doing it then you already know about its benefits. There are three main crawling exercises that can be tried out for maximum effectiveness; the bear crawling movement, the spider crawling movement, and the grok crawling movement.

-Single side exercises and levers

If you are familiar with the lever, you might know that it is a grueling position to do. But once you can do it, it can be turned into something very interesting. It is actually an n amazing core training exercise.

It is suggested by experts that for better results, one can combine the levers and the single side exercises.

-Throwing

Yes, the power that can be generated from a simple throwing exercise can do wonders. It is an effective and easy activity that can stimulate power through the core.

There is one very good core exercise that involves throwing and it is called a kettlebell swing.

You can use any kind of an object; medicine or a slam ball, or if you want to challenge yourself, go for a kettleball. The best way to carry out the throwing exercise would be to get a friend or a partner, who will throw and catch the object that you wish to involve in the exercise. You can also do this alone and yourself will judge your throwing power judged by far you could throw the object.

The throws in the exercise should be at the level of the chest, use the legs as a primary source of power to throw, while the arm movements should just be there to direct the object. Try to do a swing throw with the object as well, because with this the object

---

will be at swung from between the legs. This is a position that extracts more power from the hips and lower abdominal area.

The core stability and strength training may not be appealing as crunches or doing lifting exercises. But know that the core strength and stability is the base of all exercises and not just the ones in core conditioning. They will go long way in making a person feel active, more ready and challenge themselves in doing more high intensity training exercises.

If you are doing these core stabilizing activities, then automatically the effect on the core will be very prominent. You will see the difference in your body and your bones as well. Your posture will be much better and you will be able to feel better about your health as well.

Chapter 4

Core Conditioning After Pregnancy

Most women who have just had a baby are overwhelmed with the changes in their bodies. It has been much talked about how much pressure women are under to get their pre pregnancy bodies back again. Regardless of how many women have spoken about how unfair it is to expect that new mothers will go right back to looking as they were before, the thought still remains.

The media surely does not help in easing the problem. If you look through magazines, television and the social media; you will come across many people who write in magazines, blog and speak about getting back into shape after giving birth. These people cite examples of celebrities and models who barely have any post baby weight and proudly flaunt their slim frames merely weeks or a few months after having their babies.

Do not be impressed by those, it is not really anything to worry about. Every woman has her own body type and during pregnancy have different diet and exercise plans. So if you are worried about how a model has managed to look so fabulous and why you are still sporting a tummy pouch, do not be bothered.

Even if you are a woman who has exercised during the pregnancy and have done lifting as well, there can be that tummy coming out. The muscles that used to be toned and were the abs before the pregnancy are responsible for that. Usually for most women, these muscles become loose and do not function well at all. They have been stretched and battered during the pregnancy and will take a lot of time to get back to their position.

Loose muscles in this core area mean low strength. You will be able to feel the effects of these muscles very shortly. You will start experiencing back pains from picking up little weights and even holding your baby sometimes. The abdominal muscles have little or no function, and this means that the back muscles are putting in double the effort to support the lower abdominal area and torso.

There is even more pressure on the lower abdominal area since the upper body has increased the pressure. Simply put, the extra weight of the breasts pulls down on it and weighs the back muscles even further.

Needless, to say if you have been following the book closely you have now realized that the core area does not just mean abs, there are other muscles that are just as much important. These muscles make up the entire midsection area, along with the back and hips.

Pregnancy affects each and every one of those areas that encompass your core. The abdominal muscles have already been stretched and overworked; the back muscles are weakening and weighing down with all the extra work they have to out in, while the hips also are not very supportive anymore.

Many women talk about their body changes and state how their exercise routines take a major hit after pregnancy. Due to all the muscular weakening, they are unable to attempt any rigorous routine, and many also just quit doing it altogether. This is where the mistake lies.

You only have to reconnect with core, if you are woman who has been eating healthy, doing regular exercise and maintained a proper lifestyle then there should be no problem in doing that. The strength in the core is still there, you just have to find it and stimulate it through the body again.

The only problem with the core is that it is losing its ability to maintain the required intra-abdominal pressure that is needed to keep the torso straight in position and erect. Since it can no longer do that efficiently, you have been experiencing pains, lethargy and a dullness that is hampering your everyday functioning.

This is when one should seriously get up and take control again. Rebuild the core before the damage becomes too extensive and you are left with a weak core area, less stability and weakness.

Start with the basics and the get on to lifting heavy weights.

-Diastasis Recti

This is a pretty common condition; however it can become dangerous for so women if it gets severe. Assess your condition properly to know if you diastasis recti. This usually happens when the connective abdominal muscle tissue that is found in the upper abdominal region, begin to thin. This eventually causes the muscles to separate.

To check if you have the condition of diastasis recti, just lie on the back. Contract the abdominal muscles and then press lightly and gently into the abdomen below and above the navel.

If there is a soft gap or spot between the muscles, then there is indeed a separation. If the gap or space is about one to two finger widths then that is fine and you do not have to worry much. The gap will close on its own. However, if it is wider then try consulting a physical therapist on how to close the gap and restrict the muscles again.

-Symphysis Pubis Dysfunction

This is quite a painful condition and some women are known to experience it during pregnancy. The symphysis pubis dysfunction or SPD as it can be called can occur after giving birth. When a woman suffers from this SPD, it simply means that the ligaments that are responsible for keeping the pelvis aligned have become lax or loose. This eventually leads to instability in the pelvic joint, and allow it move freely and now how it is intended to move.

It is painful, not only that, it can seriously affect a person's physical movements and affect their workout routines after pregnancy, sometimes during as well. Any kind of a workout, squats, pistol squats and lunges or anything too strenuous can leave a person writhing in excruciating pain.

There is another condition called post-partum pelvic pain that can develop in some women after one or two pregnancies.

This is a condition that results in consistent or frequent pelvic pain. Because of that, even something as simple as running can hurt. It is best to consult a physical therapist and follow their instructions, the problem usually lie within the hip area and lower abdomen. Exercises like pelvic tilts, abdominal bracing and a few others can go a long way with helping the muscles gain strength again.

Now that we have discussed the possible problems that can arise in physical movements due to pregnancy, let's discuss a few easy exercise remedies. These exercises are focused on working the transverse abdominal and the pelvic floor muscles that are the base of a strong core. The exercises are easy enough that anyone can do them soon after having a baby. For women who have had a caesarean, it is advised that they wait a little while or they can risk damaging the tissues and opening the incision.

To prepare for such exercises, include the belly breathing exercises, pelvic tilts and abdominal bracing in the daily routine as soon as possible after birth. Add the arm and leg bracing movements as well to get the abdomen ready for a more intense workout.

These are some of the core exercises that can be good for new mothers. Isometric abdominal exercises are the most crucial and should be done for the first few months after the baby has been delivered.

There is the American College of sports medicine that tried to figure out which abdominal exercises were the best for reactivating the obliques and rectus abdominus. Researchers found that the yoga poses such as yoga boat, yoga dolphin plank on a ball and the yoga side plank are the most effective of exercises that can help with stimulating these muscles again.

Some of the exercises below are what have been found to be included in the conclusions of the research as well.

-Belly Breathing

As evident by the name, the belly breathing is an exercise that is simply about breathing. While doing this, let the muscles in the stomach contract and expand with inhaling and exhaling movements respectively. Try to inhale and exhale as deeply as possible.

-Abdominal bracing

Begin by lying on the floor face up. Race the abdomen by contracting all the muscles in the region, like if you are preparing to get punched or hit in the stomach. This is the starting position, then go on to movements that are varied. Raise one or two arms over the head or extend the legs while keeping the back flat against the floor.

-Pelvic Tilt

Lie on the back with the knees bent and feet flat against the ground or use a ball to prop yourself. Brace the abdomen and tilt the pelvis backwards by pressing the lower back in the floor. Try to hold the position for five seconds and then repeat.

-Yoga boat

Start by sitting on the floor with the knees bent. Brace the abdomen, the slightly lean back with your torso while lifting the feet off from the floor. Keep on lifting till the shins are parallel to the ground, the back is straight and the hips are flexed to almost ninety degrees.

The arms should be extended forward, till a comfortable position is maintained that can help you keep the balance. Hold that position for at least up to thirty seconds.

-Dolphin Plank

This sounds interesting fun and might even turn out to be. Place the elbows on top of a stability ball and extend the legs out from behind. Then brace the muscles of the abdominal region and the hips, keep the back as straight as you can and hold on to that position for half a minute at least.

It is like doing a plank, only more interesting. There is stability ball involved that makes the exercise fun and more effective as well.

-Side Plank

Begin this one by lying on the side with the elbows under the shoulder. Stack the hips and as well as the feet, then go on to stabilizing your core in the position, then finally try to lift the hips off the ground till the body is able to form a straight alignment in a line.

Hold the position on one side for thirty seconds, the break. Repeat on the other side for the same amount of time. If you are looking to challenge yourself further in this, try adding ten to about twenty leg shifts to the exercise of the side plank. This will also lead to an improvement in stability and core strength.

These were some of the exercises that women going through post pregnancy body changes can apply to gain back their core stability and recondition it as well.

However, most women who have just had a baby are so overwhelmed by their new responsibility and are caught up with taking care of the new arrival that they feel that they cannot really attempt all this. Is all this really necessary to getting it back?

Well, experts advise that these women can also try lifting to get back into shape. However this may take a lot of unnecessary time and effort. This is because it is very difficult to get back to lifting after having a baby, and the weights will have to be much lighter at the start till a long time.

Lifts are very effective and an excellent core exercise and you should not just give up on these because it takes time. It is just difficult at this particular time in your life since the torso is already unstable and the muscles are loosened. You will not be able to get a lot done in time and there will be constant fatigue as well. The effects will take very long to show and most women just quit midway because the effects take so long to show.

It is advised that you start light and progress slowly to more intense workouts. When you add in more core training in, you can drive up the results and see them faster than you think.

Post pregnancy there can be a lot of new problems to deal with, so do not stress yourself out thinking about toning the body and getting rid of baby weight. Even these particular exercises cannot contribute a lot to getting the pouch in the tummy in. They are there to stabilize and strengthen the core again so that people can do the high intensity workouts and weight lifting with vigor and health. These exercises will help tighten the muscles and eliminate any pain in the region so it becomes easier to train when you become ready for that.

Chapter 5
The Inner Unit

Experts describe the inner unit as an area in abdomen that all the muscle energy can be focused upon. The inner unit is simply a tern that can be used to describe the energy that functions within the muscles and between in some of the specific groups of the abdominal muscle.

The experts describe the inner unit training and conditioning as essential to the working of the body. It provides the joints with much needed stability and facilitates their stiffness so that they can give the prime movers in the body a good, solid working foundation.

The unit can be looked at as a stabilizing agent in the muscular formation and it can act as a protection to the internal system as well. Not only that it is also a way to control and exercise breathing, and in turn affects the autonomic nervous system. If you are able to work the inner unit effectively then that can not only lead to the stabilization of the spine but also enable the prime movers to function efficiently and get their job done. It also helps with the abilities to breath and move.

To start with let's look over some of the researches. There are a number of exercises that can focus upon the abdominal muscles, some say even a hundred. There are entire classes dedicated to working upon the completely wearing out the abdominal muscles of a person. There are exercises such as leg raise, side band and intense crunches that can work with training these abdominal muscles.

One of the experts set out on the task of examining the relation between the abdominal exercises, body alignments, pain and the appearance of a person. The expert measured everything in great detail.

He examined the head posture that goes forward, rib cage posture, pelvic tilt and the complete posture alignment. He realized that the results showed that the people who were doing the high intensity crunching and sit up exercises were having no effect on any body movements. Similarly, people who were attending the 'ab blasts' classes or indulging in high powered abdominal workout routines had a difficult time in overcoming the back aches and did not experience that much of an improvement in posture or body alignment.

The expert studied a lot of people and deduced that there was a direct link between the abdominal muscles and exercise routines. Almost a ninety-eight percent of them who complained of back pains and weakness had very less strength in their abdominal muscles as well as the transverse abdominis muscles. Those who had no such history or any sort of back pain were able to generate better strength and activation in their transverse abdominis muscles and were able to coordinate their abdominal muscles and stability better.

For the people who had backaches and any such complaints, the expert suggested that they remain away completely from any sort of crunching or sit up exercises. And he reported the people who adhered to his advice, experienced immediate improvement. They were able to witness a decrease or complete elimination of the back pains and as they exercised with other routines progressively, they also saw their posture and alignment improve significantly.

The expert analyzed research from other experiments as well observed that their conclusion that developed a relation between the back and abdominal muscles. They deduced that these muscles were functioning together as one unit. The abdominal wall that is deep within works with the other muscles such as oblique and transverse abdominis and form the inner unit.

The inner unit is different from the outer one. This expert notes that the inner unit is under a separate neurological control than the external obliques and outer rectus abdominis. Traditional gym workouts and training routines are not really that effective in activating and stimulating the functions of the muscles in the inner unit. Their ability to improve the spine movement and stability will not experience any enhancement until there is better and automatic control of the reflexes.

To attain a better and automatic reflex control among the muscles and functioning in the inner unit, it is suggested that one tries specific isolation training and build upon the sensory and motor control. Once the control is undertaken, the inner unit movements must be incorporated in to most of the daily functioning of an individual. This is because if the inner unit conditioning is not thorough and very specific, it can be hazardous to the health sometimes. Sometimes people have stated that their spinal movements are unstable and can even incur spine injury.

Going in to further detail if one wants to know the science of the inner unit, one can look towards Paul Chek's explanation of the term. He described it as being the 'functional synergy' between the muscles of the pelvic floor, transverse abdominis, obliquus internus abdominis and lumbar parts. The diaphragm is involved in the inner unit as well.

It is under a different neurological control than the other core muscles that explains why such exercises which focused on the abdominal muscles and rectus abdominis were of little to no use in getting the spine in its stable position and reducing the back pains.

The bigger muscles, which are the prime movers and their exercises, were not providing the right strength and foundation to the small muscles such as pelvic floor and transverse abdominis.

When these muscles are functioning properly and at full capacity, the muscles give stiffness to joints, and stability to the spine. The rib cage and pelvis muscles provide a strong and stable foundation for the big muscles. It is said that the more tighter and stronger the big muscles, they can cause a disruption in the balance between the inner and outer unit.

If you want a better understanding of the functioning between the inner and outer unit, try picking up dumbbells off the floor. When the thought goes into the mind, the brain automatically activates the inner unit. Such tasks require a synergistic coordination and functioning between the inner and outer units. If the inner unit is weak and fails to get activated at the right time, the spinal movements can be disrupted. This can lead to spine injury or even joint injuries.

Other than that if you fail to produce an effective inner and outer unit synergy, there can other repercussions as well. Many gym instructors and people focus the core training upon the creation of six packs. This is dangerous. As reiterated a couple of times in the previous chapters as well, do not just focus the core training on the abs and six pack building. Here it will disrupt the inner unit functioning and lead to core stability imbalance as well. People might experience distorted breathing patterns, bad posture, no body alignment and problems with joint.

To maintain an efficient inner unit core function, the first step to take is to stop all the crunches and sit up exercises completely. This will reduce the back pains; improve posture and the overall appearance as well. Begin with the very basic exercises, even the athletes who are into advance training should begin from novice levels. The reason why many people in this day and age do not have efficient core and inner unit function is because they do not focus properly on the right kind of exercises.

Begin by conditioning the transverse abdominis. The exercise for that is a four point transverse abdominis trainer. For other muscles and stabilizing there are the horse stance exercises that could help give a person a better posture. These are just a few of the exercises available for the inner unit; there are many others that can work as well. If they are done the right way, these exercises can go a long way in making the inner unit function effectively. And you yourself will be able to feel the difference.

-Four Point Transverse Abdominis Trainer

Start with a crouching position, where the knees are touching the ground and the upper body is lifted above on both hands. The palms of the hands should be flat against the floor.

When you have maintained the spine in neutral alignment, allow the belly to drop towards the floor. Then exhale and draw the navel in, as far as you can, towards the spine. Once the air has been let out, try and hold the navel in towards the spine for as much time as you can, without breathing in or taking any breath.

Through the breathing pattern, keep the spine straight and motionless. Repeat the process at least ten times and complete the set.

You can rest till up to a minute after completing a single set. When you have done that, you will be able to build up enough strength to do three sets of the routine. It is advised that for maximum results, you must do this at least two to three times.

-Horse Stance

Vertical:

Place the wrists right below the shoulders and have your knees below the respective hip joint. The legs should be kept parallel and the elbows should be positioned facing back towards thighs, with the fingers pointing forward.

Take the help of a dowel rod to position the spine in perfect alignment. The rod should be facing the floor. The space that is between the lower back and the rod should be measured to about a thickness of the hand. The alignment is very important.

Draw the navel in towards the spine, just enough that a space is created.

It is suggested that you take help from or assistant from someone who can better judge the alignment of the spine and its position. If you are unable to find anyone, take help from mirrors. Train in an area with large mirror and see the alignment for yourself.

The horse stance vertical is started by lifting just one hand off the floor, just enough so that a very minute space is created between them. The space should be enough for a sheet of paper to slide through, not more than that. The knee that is opposite to the hand should be lifted off for that much space as well. During this movement, ensure that the level of the rod is maintained and the alignment is proper. Hold the position for about ten seconds and then change sides. Life the other hand and knee just enough to let a paper slide between those and the floor or a mat if you are using one.

The optimum number of repetitions for each of these movements is ten on each side, the position also being held for ten seconds. When you can successfully attempt three sets of the exercise with a minute break between them, then you are ready to incorporate this in your daily exercise program.

There are other horse stance exercises as well.

The start position for all of the horse stance exercise is the same. Crouch and elevate the upper body with the help of your hands. The knees should be on the ground.

Raise an arm to at least forty five degrees off the midline area and hold them in the exact horizontal plane as the back. Keep the thumbs upwards so that they point out.

Lift the leg opposite the arm that you have raised and take it up to the point at which the leg is in line with the horizontal plane as the torso. Try left arm and right leg combination at first and then change it as you progress further. As the leg is being elevated, try and keep the pelvis where it is. The pelvis should not be tilted and you can gauge the movement of the pelvis as the space between the lower back and the rod will increase. This can disrupt the alignment of the posture.

Try and hold the leg out straight so that the muscles in the buttocks are activated. During the exercise, at no point, should the pelvis or shoulder girdle lose their horizontal position parallel to the floor or a mat if you are using that for exercise.

It is common during these movements that the shoulders to drop on the sides of the arm that is elevated, even the hip rises sometimes on the side of the leg that is extended. If this happens then that means that your form is poor and fitness level is low.

The arm and leg are both held in their respective positions for ten seconds and then you can alternate sides. Repeat this for up to ten times on each side, if you maintain a proper alignment and form through the movements. You can keep yourself in check by getting help from a partner or using a mirror.

The exercises are fairly simple yet they are technical to do as precision and maintaining a proper alignment is essential when you are performing them. To get the optimum results from these exercises, try and doing them about three or four times a week, both as a separate workout or even as part of your training program. It is suggested that if you have any back problems or spinal ones, then just stop doing all those crunches and sit up routines. Replace them with all these ones and see the difference within yourself.

The inner unit exercise should be performed during the last segment of the exercise and training session. That is that you do each of the inner unit exercise after doing each workout.

To avoid monotony and boredom, mix up the routines a bit. Alternate each time with a four point transversus abdominis trainer or any type of the horse stance exercises that can be done after every workout or training session.

There are certain instructions also that should be followed with each exercise as failing to be precise in these sessions will make the entire effort futile.

For example during the horse stance exercise it is essential that you follow these; the head and neck should stay aligned with the spine, the head should not droop or tilt and definitely not be lifted any time. The elbow of the arm that is supporting you should be pointing directly towards the back and not to any side. The arm that is lifted up should be at an angle of forty five degrees just off the midline. The arms and shoulders should be at a level and parallel to the floor at all times. No movement should come from the lower back and if there is it should be very little. All movements should be directed towards the hips. The lower leg and the thighs should function as one unit. Keep the navel drawn in towards the spine, because otherwise there could be disruptions in the respirations.

Having a good inner unit is essential in everyday functioning. Researchers have also experimented on its relationship with breathing and they have hypothesized that increasing the strength of the inner unit can facilitate better respiration as well.

The muscles in the inner unit are also sometimes referred to as tonic muscles. The usually function as stabilizers and as you know play a vital role in stabilizing the spine, not only that they are effective in sacroiliac joint movements and reducing the levels of fatigue.

For people who wonder about that, there is an answer to that as well. It has been observed that in people who have no history or complaints of back problems, the transversus abdominis is instigated and fired up to thirty milliseconds before an arm movement and a hundred and ten milliseconds before leg movements.

When the body is activated, so is the inner unit. That results in the contraction of the transversus abdominis and multifidi. The fibres of transversus abdominis are of a horizontal orientation, and because of that the umbilicus gets drawn in towards the spine when a contraction occurs. This action of drawing in of the wall compresses the internal organs in the abdominal region. This up and down movement that occurs due to the compression of the wall against the organs is responsible for activating the diaphragm and as well as the pelvic floor muscles. This movement that occurs simultaneously as an activation of the inner unit is the cause of the stiffening of spinal cord and provides stabilization to other regions as well.

The contraction of tranversus abdominis is very important for a number of reasons; the abdominal wall that draws in when there is a transversus abdominis contraction is responsible for increasing the intra-abdominal pressure. The movement is also the main reason behind the stabilization of each vertebra. Lumbar muscles and obliquus abdominis are involved in the process which is quite complicated. The extensors in the back and multifidus combine with other muscles and produce a mechanism called the hydraulic amplifier mechanism. It is said that this mechanism is proven to be effective towards increasing the strength of the extensors in the back by up to a thirty percent.

This chapter has discussed in detail al there is to know about the inner unit. Hopefully you will be able to work upon the exercises that have been mentioned in the chapter and even find them effective. If there are persistent health problems it is advised that a person consult a doctor or a therapist before attempting to these exercises. Also be very careful about how you do them. Your form should be fit and body alignment very precise otherwise there will be no or very little effect on your health and body.

Chapter 6

Core Conditioning and Pain relief

For most people who are inactive, there can be a lot of health problems that arise due to their immobility. Core conditioning might be a solution to at least of them. Many people who are involved with sitting most of the time, experience these problems. Too much time in one position is hazardous to health, especially the back region.

The people who have desk jobs, they can spend about hours sitting in the same position. And even when they hit the gym, the exercises they might choose could just contribute in increasing the tightness in their body instead of rejuvenating the muscles and building them.

The core area is the essential area when it comes to muscle strengthening so if you are trying to find a way to easy up and work upon your back, then start from here.

Do not subject your core to the frequent spinal flexion or bicycle crunches that are so common within people after they complete their cardio. The idea is to build a very strong, almost bulletproof core, and to do that you need exercises that can help you maintain a core with strength and stability.

And to build a strong core, here are some of the exercises that you can try out.

-Standing Rope Crunch

This is just a modification of the popularly done kneeling rope crunch. This is the standing version of that and is known to be more effective than the kneeling rope crunch. It is more effective because it allow the upper and lower body to tie together while maintaining some tension in the core area. It is a good way to actually feel 'the burn' and you won't have to do fifty reps for that.

The rope should be held from a high position and then the person should step back from the cable stack. Then the hips should be pushed in the middle, like the position of a Romanian deadlift. This will be an individual's starting and ending position. Now without moving the arms draw the ribcage and pull it towards the pelvis. Hold the squeezing position for about three to two seconds and then release. Try and attempt up to fifteen or even twenty-five reps of this exercise.

-Palloff lift and press

This is one of the staple exercises for people since it is self-limiting and there is very little to almost no possibility of doing it wrong. If you are not feeling the palloff press and lift correctly, you might get pulled. You should be tight during this exercise. It is an efficient and good way to activate or re-activate the core if you did not manage to do it before. It gets you mentally prepared for it as well.

Start the exercise by standing in a perpendicular position, which is to a cable machine with the cable at almost the chest height. Now in slow and controlled movements, push it away from the body. When the cable has been completely extended, lift the arms over your head, again only in very slow and controlled movements. Bring the hand back downward in an extended position. Then take the hands back to your chest.

This is just one rep, you should do about ten to six reps of these repeated on both the sides.

-Landmine rotation and foot movement

This exercise is actually done through foot movement. It is a great exercise and helps train the core in a number of places. It will also help you stay up and braced during other dynamic movements. It actually works wonders for people involved in rotational sports like golf, throwing, kickboxing, etc.

Start by setting up a landmine or just a barbell in a corner that is sturdy. Hold the end of that by extending your hands, and then pull your ribs down. Pull them down in the front so that a bracing level is created and across all levels of core musculature.

Keep the chest up and drop the head of the barbell down, to right side. Now as you drop this down, step the left foot towards the barbell's anchor point. Do this so the toe is now facing straight towards the right, the start bringing the barbell up. Slowly bring it up without losing the tension in the core and then place the foot back to where it was when you started. Repeat the same on the opposite side. All this makes up one rep. You are advised to do at least ten reps.

-Standing ab wheel roll out

You see those models and wonder how they got those tone six pack abs, well the answer is through this exercise. Yes but other than focusing on building abs, it is a very good core strengthening exercise as well. However many do not attempt this as they cannot perform the exercise properly due to kneeling and standing differences. This should not deter people.

They can use resistance bands while starting, and as they progress further and become good at training in this advanced position, the band can be removed.

Ensure that when you are performing the exercise, you only go as far as you can maintain the spine in the neutral position or a hollow position of the body. When you comeback from the bottom which is the last position in the exercise, try fitting in a crunch in their as well. This will stress the abs further. Do at least eight to twelve abs.

-Anti Gravity Pullover

Contrary to the other exercises, this is not a standing exercise. However it will extend your body fully and maintains the spine at neutral. The exercise involves using and manipulating the gravity to boost the body with the external stimulant that is necessary to give three different resistance aspects.

This exercise works upon the anti- rotation, anti-extension and anti-lateral flexion, which are all integral components of the core. They help keep your back strong as and even give you the much coveted six packs.

Begin the exercise by placing your hips on the edge of the bench, in a way that your torso is falling off the bench. To ensure that you do not fall off, place the bottom leg in the front and then hook the heel right under the bench.

You might probably be thinking what kind of an exercise this is. Actually, it's a very interesting one.

Now take the top foot and then out it back also, with the toe hooked under the bench. From that position, locate a cable or any band that is at least five feet away from you. When you find that, pull on it. Pull that band from eye level down to the bottom of the hips, and maintain the core tension throughout the movement. Do approximately eight to ten reps on each of the sides.

These are all the exercises that can strengthen your core a great deal and help alleviate any kinds of pains as well.

Now that we have talked about core strengthening exercises, let's talk about some of their benefits as well.

A good and strong core reduces back pain substantially. The weak and unbalanced core muscles are actually what cause the back pain. The weak core muscles are what result in the loss of the lumbar curve and back posture. The stronger and balanced your core muscles are, the better will be the posture and less strain it will incur on the spine.

66

A strong core is the reason behind a good and efficient performance in athletics. The trunk muscles and torso are the stabilizing agents behind the spine, right from the pelvis to the neck and shoulders. The also facilitate the transfer of power from the arms and legs. The powerful movements of the body are originated from the center of the body and not just from the limbs alone. So before any powerful movements or rapid muscle contractions can take place, it is essential for the spine to be solid and stable. The more stable the core, the more power can be generated within the extremities.

Finally a good core is responsible for improving postural imbalances. When you train the core muscles, it automatically helps improve the posture that could possibly result in injuries. One of the biggest benefits of training the core is to attain a functional fitness level. It also improves health that is much needed in everyday life activities as well and not just in athletics.

To strengthen the core it is essential that you work upon the torso and back movements as well. They are the most effective when there is an integration of multi joints movements, front muscles and back muscles, along with the torso as well. It must work as one unit. Stabilization of the spine should also be monitored during the strength training.

You already are aware of the abdominal bracing that is necessary to follow before all such exercises.

Exercises that efficiently combine all the above mentioned movements would be planks, side planks, v-sits, pushups and supermans among others.

Athletes have also complained about the back pain that comes from these exercises and the reason for that is that their core muscles are weak when it comes to the sport they are playing. Some may just experience spinal pain and other things due to injury.

For them also it is advised that they should not just rush into alleviating the pain. The should first start by building the strength of their core areas and muscles and then go towards the challenging and grueling core conditioning exercises once the strength has been maintained.

For athletes the main problem can arise in the lower back area. It is one of main strength producing areas in any field. Whether it is the track or swimming pool, the lower back is one of the essential components of the body in any sporting activity.

The lower back is what channels the power and energy from the body and optimizes the core. It also provides protection against any spinal injuries or such. To indulge in athletic activities properly, it is essential that one has a very strong lower back.

The more essential this area is to the athletic functioning, the more prone it is to weakening of muscles and deficiencies. It is quite common for athletes to complain about their lower back areas and injuries in the region. Working on one part of the spine could produce the weakness in the muscles. This can create an imbalance that can even injure the lower back. Even if one area in the lower back is weak, the effects will be felt everywhere and ultimately can lead to weakening of the entire region.

Think of it like links in a chain, each link has to depend on the other for support. Even if one is weak or missing the entire chain collapses. Same is the case here.

The most common back injuries are found in Olympic athletes. They are the one who generally report having low back problems and sometimes even have to pull out of competitions due to that. Especially among athletes who are in lifting competitions.

The extra strain, stress and weights on this part of the body according to the demand of the competition makes it essential for the lifter to have a strong core and low back. The lifter's motion is of a wide range and requires that the core be strong to carry them efficiently and also prevent any injury.

Sometime athletes may deliberately choose to ignore this part of the body, like the back, the glutes or the hamstrings simply due to vain reasons. These parts of the body are not that prominent when it comes to display and the other such as abs and stomach get noticed more often. Hence the athletes might just skip the exercises and neglect the area.

Once they pay a much deeper notice to the area and start training properly, they themselves will notice the difference in their body and functioning that will be experienced as training these parts. The better the form of the lower back, the more efficient and smooth will be the sporting activities such as swimming, racing, sprinting or any others as well. The power in the movements will be felt more vibrantly and the body will be able to life quicker, have a quicker reflex, adapt faster, as well as be stabilized. All these functions are not just restricted to sporting activities but also essential in everyday life activities.

There are a few ways in which you strengthen your lower back and core as well. These are divided in to two categories, one of that is the dynamic stretching and the other is strength work.

The strength work includes dead lifts and squats.

During the deadlifts, focus should be on keeping the core and the lats very tight during the progression of the exercise. Only the movement of the legs is the focus and not the entire body. The legs also pull very slowly. The deadlift is one of the most effective exercises that can help with maintaining a healthy lower back.

Squats are of course, responsible for developing the glutes and upper thighs, as well as the low back. A good and proper squat begins with the heels no further apart than distance or width between the hips while the toes are angled to approximately thirty or twenty degrees. Bend yourself at the waist a little, but maintain the back in as flat a way as you can. Look straight ahead and not upwards as you are bending around the knees, putting pressure on the heels. As you are rising up, work up the glutes and other muscles such as hamstrings. Be careful that the back does not get rounded up.

The important aspect of maintaining and keep on building a strong low back being aware of the area at every time. That does not mean that you pay less attention to other areas. Focus on the spine and the other abdominal muscles as well. Make sure that you concentrate on all the core muscles and try to work upon them as a unit.

You will feel the effects of them not just on one area but upon your overall health and lifestyle as well.

Konrad Obidoski

Chapter 7

Core Conditioning Exercises Just for Women

For women there are specific exercises just based on the core. If they are looking to get a six pack or tone up their stomach, the core is where they should put most of their focus. For women who are already doing Pilates and go to the gym regularly, working on the core will be easy.

It will be slightly difficult for women who do not go to the gym or have desk jobs that require little movement. The midsection is one where that is of a huge concern among women. That and the glutes are first one that gain weight and prominently show the gain as well. Due to this tendency of bloating women worry about keeping their stomach toned a lot.

It does not help that the media has created these unrealistic ideals of how a woman's body should be. This just increases the pressure for most women to look in shape, especially during and after pregnancy.

The most efficient and fastest way to tone down the bulge in the stomach is to hit the core area. Working all these muscles will surely take off inches from the midsection and help women gain a slimmer, tiny waist.

To do these core exercises, it is essential to first strengthen the core.

Here are a few ways in which that can be done.

-Knee fold tuck

This is fairly easy to do. Just sit tall, keep your hands in the floor and squeeze a playground ball in between them. Then lift the knees so that the shins are parallel to the floor and then extend the arms. Pull the knees towards the shoulders and keep the upper body still. Then bring the knees back to the starting position. Repeat that for about fifteen to twenty times.

-Climbing the rope

First sit with the legs extended in the front and then turn your feet out into a V position. The toes should be pointed out. Contract the core muscles and then roll the spine in to a C-curve. Lift the arms and move them up as if you were climbing a rope. Twist slightly every time you reach for it. Attempt at least twenty reaches with one each arm.

-Side balance crunch

Begin with the left knee and left hand placed on the floor. Keep the right arm straight up. Extend the right leg in a way that the body forms a straight line.

Then pull the right knee towards the torso, and the right elbow towards the knee; then straighten both the arms and legs. Repeat at least ten times on one side and then switch the sides.

-Circle Plank

Start this one in a plank position, keeping your abs tight. Pull the right knee in and then circle it clockwise. After that, also move it counter clockwise.

Make sure that the rest of the body is stationary. Repeat up to five times and then switch the legs.

-Sliding the pike

Try to do this movement on an uncarpeted surface. Begin in a position of the plank, with the hands right under the shoulders. Keep a towel underneath your feet.

While keeping your legs straight, raise the hips and draw the legs in towards the hands in a pike position. Because of the towel, your feet should be able to slide easily. Hold for one single count and then return to the starting position. Repeat this at least ten times.

-Oblique Reach

You must sit straight with your knees bent and feet on the floor. Straighten the right leg, and roll the spine into a C-curve. Place the left hand behind the head and extend the right arm. Twist the body to the left side and try to roll back slightly more. Hold for a second in that position and the release. You can come up then. Do five reps and then switch sides.

These were some of the easy ways to try and strengthen the core. They are very effective as well. Once you are able to do these properly, you will feel the difference in the core area yourself and will feel much stronger and healthier.

Once the core has been strengthened, you can move towards the intense workouts that will include abs toning and stomach reducing as well.

The main aspect of core training and working with high intensity core exercises is to not just restrict yourself to crunches. While crunches are effective in ab building, they will not have that much effect on reducing the tummy pouch that almost all women aim to get rid of.

The crunch works with only one part of the core and that is just not done, because, it will not be of much use if you are trying to maintain a slim waistline. To reduce the size of your stomach you must try and work with the entire core muscle, which includes the hip muscles, flexors and glutes as well. The lower back is also of much importance and all the other ab muscles as well; such as, rectus abdominis, obliques, and the very crucial one which is the transversus abdominis. You must remember that these muscles should be worked upon from every angle and not just from the front to back, like with crunches.

The following exercises will focus upon all the muscles and not just the singular motions. These routines are more effective than just sculpting your six pack and those muscles, they engage almost all the muscles in the core region and even increase the fat burning power of the body.

The exercises here will not only work the work but also help with the toning of arms and legs, increase strength in the shoulder and chest muscles, and just boost the overall health of the body.

-Kettlebell windmill

Its core target is the obliques or the side abs.

Take hold of a kettlebell with the left hand and then stand with the feet more than the hip width apart. Then bring the weight next to the left shoulder, and press it over the head. Rotate the chest to the left and look up to the kettlebell as you are doing that, while you can also try and touch the right foot with the right hand. Pause for a moment, then return to start. Keep the left arm extended while you do.

Do almost eight reps of this and then lower the weight. After that, switch to the other side.

-Swiss ball jackknife

The area of the core that this targets is the transversus abdominis or lower abs.

You have to use a stability ball for this workout. Get in to a pushup position with the arms straight ahead and the shins resting on the stability ball. Then roll the ball towards the chest by using the feet and legs to pull it forward. Pause for a while and then return to your starting position. When you do that, you should lower the hips while also pushing the ball backwards with the legs. Do about ten reps of this and you will see great results.

-Unsupported one arm row

The core target of this routine is the rectus abdominus, or the area the build upon the six pack. It also helps and strengthens the obliques.

Hold a kettlebell in the right hand and place the top of the left hand on the lower back and then stand with your feet at least shoulder width apart. Lower the torso until it's almost parallel to the floor and keep the back flat and knees bent slightly. Let your arm hang from the shoulder and then pull the weight to the side of your chest. Do not move the torso while you are doing this. Pause and then lower the weight back to the start. Do at least eight reps and then repeat from the left side.

-The rolling side planks

The target of this is the rectus abdominis, the obliques and transversus abdominis.

Start in the plank position, forearms should be on the ground and legs should be extended behind. Then rotate your torso to the side, roll on to the forearm to the left and stack your right foot on the top of your left in the position of a side plank. Hold on to that position for one or two seconds, and then return to the starting position. Hold on for one second and then repeat on the other side. Continue to alternate sides for at least forty-five seconds.

Complete all these exercises in a circuit by progressing through each one without taking a break. Start with at least four circuits to maximize results and then rest for about sixty to ninety seconds in between each set. If you want to take this up a notch, increase the circuits and lower the resting time.

Since most women feel that it is a challenge to lose all the tummy fat, they try harder. And if you are willing to see these results, you should be willing to work hard as well.

There are experts who have described other exercises that can be very efficient in core building and weight losing. Doing about five to ten sets of these, three or four times a week can produce wondrous results on the body.

-The ball roll out

There have been tests done that show that even the most inactive muscles get fired up during this exercise. The hips muscles have very less involvement in this exercise so there is very less chance of an injury. This exercise is really good for new mothers as it helps with the alignment and body posture as well.

Kneel behind a large exercise ball and place your arms on top of it. Extend the hands and keep them very straight. Begin rolling the ball slowly away from you, while stretching the body out as you go. Roll out as far out as you can without losing balance and control of the ball.

-Pilates Beginner 100

Lie on the back and bend your knees, keeping your feet together. Lift the bend legs away from the floor and align your knees with the hips. Stretch the arms out at the side, just a few inches above the floor. The palms should be facing downwards. Towards the spine, pull in the belly button.

One of the other effective exercises in here is the side plank. That works very effectively on the core as well. It is also responsible for preventing the spine into bending in a C-shape.

-The yoga beginner boat

This one works upon the obliques and the abdominal muscles.

Begin by sitting up tall on the floor, with the legs straight outwards and the palms facing down. The fingertips should be pointed towards the feet. Try to keep the spine tall and still lifted while you try leaning back, balance on the sit bones. Try lifting the legs as high form the floor as you can and feel comfortable with. Use the fingertips to attain balance, and bend the knees a little bit. The position of the knees should be as much as you can accommodate according to the level of strength and your fitness.

Lift the arms up so that the fingertips are kept along the knees.

You should try and hold this pose for about ten counts, as you focus on staying upright and keeping the chest lifted up as well.

-The pilates double stretch

This works effectively for aging women. The benefits of this exercise are shown in the women as it helps reduces the tummy sags and pouch efficiently.

Lie on the back and pull the belly button towards the spine. Bring in your knees towards the chest and take hold of your shins firmly. Now round up the back to lift your head, and then the neck and shoulders off the ground. Take a deep breath and inhale while extending your legs out straight, at least a foot of the floor. Now stretch the arms behind you so that the elbows are along the side of the ears.

Exhale deeply and sweep the arms around in a circle, and pull the knees back towards the chest.

These are some of the exercises that work very efficiently in producing the desired results on the stomach and abs.

If women start practicing these daily or even weekly, they will see the prominent results as soon as they can. Just doing these exercises will not help; you will also have to eat right with these exercises. Maintain a healthy lifestyle. Avoid soda drinks or fizzy drinks. Keep away from alcohol. If you can, consult a nutritionist or dietician to maintain a healthy lifestyle.

Do not indulge in too many fatty foods; a reason for tummy pouch is the collection of fat that is of course through eating too many carbs.

Eat more greens and vegetables, while keeping away from the harmful foods that can affect your health and render all the exercise useless.

Eating healthy:

It is one of the most integral parts of maintaining a good health. This goes for men and women both. They must not just rely on the core conditioning exercises to keep toned up. Along these exercises, it is essential that they eat healthy and take the right nutrition as well.

Start by taking a healthy and nutritious breakfast. Take lots of proteins and natural juices. If you are a regular coffee drinker, then cutting down on the amount of caffeine is also suggested.

Use fiber and dietary fibers, and try to eat organic food. I know what I am saying sounds difficult, but if you set a resolve then you can actually try and achieve this.

After all core conditioning is all about setting goals and being determined to see them through. Crunches, sit ups and other high intensity core workouts such as dragon flag and cable chop are very meticulous and require a lot of focus and strength. In fact the dragon flag is one exercise that has been promoted by both Bruce Lee and Sylvester Stallone.

If you decide to indulge in such training, you must also keep up the food intake to match this. If you are taking in healthy and good food, then you will see exemplary results and such positive body changes within yourself.

When you start your exercise regime, you must consult a medical expert if you want. When you go to one, try and find out about your metabolism and hormone levels. You can make your meal plans according to that.

If you are a regular gym goer, chances are that your metabolism is high. That means that the rate of digestion in your body is much faster. For such people, it is advised that they try out eating throughout the day, meals of small portions and can include the good carbohydrates in their meals.

Yes, there is a difference between the good and bad carbs. The good ones can actually boost up your carb levels and stimulate better nutrition circulation in your body. You can take them with dietary fibers and incorporate it into the diet plan that you follow daily.

Women who are pregnant or have gone through pregnancy are already aware of taking the right kind of food. However there are cravings and other factors that can lead up to the weight gain in pregnancy. For some women this baby weight can be a real problem, try how hard they might, the baby weight just does not go away. Core exercises have already been suggested for that. Along with those, they should also focus on taking a protein based diet. It is healthy for the baby as well.

Pregnant women should also take lots of proteins and mineral in their diet.

It is advised that people, who train regularly, always keep themselves hydrated and drink lots of water.

Having a diet plan does not mean that a person cannot indulge occasionally. One or two cheat meals a week or on a monthly basis will not do any harm. So yes you can go all those burgers and French fries once in a while, but do remember to work extra hard after that as you will need to work off those calories.

Konrad Obidoski

Chapter 8
Core Facts and Myths

We'll get into some facts and myths that surround abdominal training. As it's one of the most sexy and trendy topics in the fitness world and in general as we approach summer, it managed to hoard a whole lot of legends while eluding facts. It probably stems from its profitability that attracts scams, but not only them. Usually people mean well – they just don't know any better.

Without further ado, let's get to the MYTHS.

Ab Myth #1 – Core equals abs

The term "core" has been dragged in the mud, torn apart, slapped and kicked and overall overused-as-hell. Core has been equated with abdominals while it is basically everything that is not your extremities, your limbs. However, for the sake of simplicity and training programming it is best to understand the core as your neck, hips (hip flexors, glutes...) and lower torso, INCLUDING your low-back. Many people tend to forget that if you train only the front of your body, the part you see in the mirror, the back part will suffer, sometimes with painful consequences.

Ab Myth #2 - Training abs everyday

For some odd reason the abdominals has been categorized separately from every other muscle group of the human body. I am not even mentioning the It is totally unnecessary and even detrimental to train your core every day. You have your chest days and your back days, your training days and your off days. Muscles grow and get stronger while they are recovering, they need that time off to rebuild, thus granting you your hard-earned gains. Training muscles every day, especially those with mostly stabilizing role will gradually de-train them to the point where you can snap your back trying to tie your shoes or you can't train any longer due to the pain you are experiencing. This is especially prevalent as for most people "core training" is doing lots and lots of crunches, which will bring us to the next myth.

Ab Myth #3 – Doing ONLY crunches

As "core" equals "abs", crunches are the only exercise you will ever need. This is a very bad thinking pattern for the reasons mentioned above. Of course crunches have their uses, however they should be the exercise used last on the list and as of now they are heavily overused, if not used exclusively by many. To achieve proper balance of muscles that will boost performance and relieve pain in most instances, one needs to train the whole abdominal area. Lower abs, upper abs, transversus abdominis and the obliques, both internal and external. And that not even mentioning the neck and back. Make everything as simple as possible, but never simpler!

Ab Myth #4 – Doing 100 crunches

Every ab training program I've ever encountered (and tried, mind you. I too was confused and didn't know any better back in the day) was built around the concept of volume work. Doing dozens of sit-ups, hundreds of crunches and working yourself up to fifty leg-raises, all unnecessary. Abdominals are phasic muscles, meaning that they are more suited for movement instead of statically keeping the body in alignment and therefore respond much better to fast-twitch muscle fibers training. Doing more than twelve repetitions will move you further into the endurance training, while abs will respond optimally to more of a strength focused training.

Ab Myth #5 – Training abs will make it less fat

People still believe that doing crunches is the only and single cause of a ripped six-pack. Even though many coaches and athletes have been beating this dead horse, the message still cannot get through. You CAN'T reduce fat on a spot. You must control your diet and exercise regularly to get to low enough body-fat percentage to allow your abdominal muscles to shine through!

Chapter 9

Basic Functional Anatomy of the Core and Training Considerations

Now you know that it is imperative to understand how your trunk is constructed and how to use it properly in order to achieve superior athletic performance and relieve any back pain you might suffer from. In this chapter we will briefly cover the most important muscles, their function and application of this information in your training. If you don't give a damn about this kind of information that you're probably not serious enough about your development or healing to truly change anything. Learn about your body enough to provide it with the right type of movement for your goals.

Neck

The neck will be probably a weak point for most of you, for most of us, really. In your neck you have important muscles, the deep flexors that are there to tilt your head forward or keep it aligned when you lie on your back. As the general population people are sitting too much, slouching and extending their neck like turtles to keep their eyes leveled, usually to see the screen. It is imperative that you balance neck muscles with the rest of your body if you want to have a stable and injury-free neck.

First step towards that goal will be learning the proper physiological position of the tongue that will define the correctness of your neck training. Swallow and notice how the tongue rests on the roof of the mouth. That's where you want to keep it during all core exercises, basically all demanding exercises. Next, you would want to see whether you need to create balance between your abs and your neck muscles. Perform a couple of crunches (remember about the tongue) with your fingers gently touching the back of your ears. Your neck will probably be fatigued after couple of reps, some of you may even experience a total inability to lift your head up with your torso.

Most likely, you will also notice that when holding your head you could bang out many more repetitions – that is an indication of an functional imbalance. However, the fix is easy. From now on, every time you are crunching or do other abdominal work, stop when exhaustion of your neck muscles would cause form breakdown.

Rectus Abdominis

Ah, yes. The famous six pack muscle. Maybe the most esthetically pleasing and overused muscle of the whole human body. It's function is to flex the trunk, to bend it forward. There are two things that are critical to understand about it. First, it must be perceived as two separate units in terms of training: lower and upper. This is important because your lower abs is responsible for stabilizing your pelvis and preventing it from tilting forward, while the upper part mostly pulls you into pronation, causing poor posture. I am not saying that the upper part is bad and shouldn't be exercised, but most people would benefit more from stretching it instead of training.

Second, the classic floor crunch allows you only to bend forward, preventing any extension, so you train with a very reduced range of motion. Did you know that your muscles are divided into units along their length, called the sarcomeres. Whenever you don't utilize full range of motion, your muscles reduce their numbers and thus effectively reduce their length. Shortened abs will constantly pull you forward causing poor posture and compromising any athletic results and possibly cause injuries down the road. Therefore, always try to use the biggest range of motion possible (just be smart, you don't have to force it). To achieve that, crunch on a swissball or any similar object to allow support yet with the ability to extend fully.

Obliques

Obliques are the, well, oblique muscles of your abdominal area that are mostly responsible for bending your trunk sideways and rotating it. They are also the main stabilizing agent whenever you have to counter any rotational force. This is important to remember, because in every time you fall or get pushed you must use your obliques to counter the force and protect your spine. Combative and other high-impact sports athletes should view this as a crucial element of their development. Moreover, every time you throw something like a ball, a javelin, a Frisbee, you use mostly rotational force channeled from your legs and core while your upper body contribute much less to the throw. From an aesthetical point of view, if you want to get that V-taper going, you have to develop your obliques.

Transversus abominis

The most neglected muscle. It is the transverse, horizontal tube that encircles your lower torso and squeezes you spine to provide maximum stability. This is the muscle you need to train, to become strong and stable. You can't train it directly, however. This is the muscle that get activated when you pull your bellybutton towards your spine and create more intra-abdominal pressure. It will be an important concept later in the text and I will further elaborate on it.

Psoas, the hip flexors

The huge muscles that pull your legs towards your stomach, bending you at the hips are also extremely important, especially that they are often overused. Remember the concept of sarcomere number decreasing as muscle is shortened? Now think how much you sit with your thighs perpendicular to your torso. What is more, have you ever did leg raises or sit-ups for "your abs"? What you did was training mostly your hip flexor with abdominals being just the stabilizing muscles. Again, I am not saying that some muscles shouldn't be trained. Try to feel the little bones sticking out of your pelvis on its front and back – these are the iliac spines. When you stand, they should be on the same level and you should have a little bit of an arch (lordosis) in your lower back. If your front iliac spines are lower and your arch is exaggerated, you definitely need to stretch the hip flexors and train the rest of your flexor chain to be equally strong and only then integrate them by doing whole flexor chain exercises.

Quadratus Lumborum

Last but not least is the quadratus lumborum, huge muscle in your loins. It pulls your pelvis forward, just like the hip flexors. When you have the opposite problem and your butt is tucked under, remember to us some back extension exercises. If you do a back extension exercise, have your front iliac spines on the bench. This will stabilize the pelvis and make your low back work to the exclusion of glutes and hamstrings. Same as with the former examples, you first want to achieve balance in strength between individual links of the chain and then integrate them to work in concert with each other.

Chapter 10

Training Techniques and Important Notions

We must discuss some important points about training your core and using it properly in movements that do not focus on its development but rely heavily on it. We'll talk about intra-abdominal pressure, breathing properly that may prove tricky to a lot of people and the usage of both in your training.

Intra-abdominal pressure

When you want a stable base to do anything, you must get tight and I mean, real tight. Did you know that shoulder-stabilizing muscles could generate as much as the equivalent of 200 pounds of pressure on your shoulder socket to keep all the bones in place when you perform, say, a throw? Why elite weightlifters sometimes prepare for minutes before a single lift? They need to be focused to use perfect technique and keep their whole body flexed to the limit to achieve maximal tightness and stability.

Your transversus abdominis muscle is mostly responsible for getting you that intra-abdominal pressure. To achieve it, take a deep breath and pull your bellybutton towards your spine. Note that you don't need to flex your abs, though it will happen as the loads get heavy enough. To perform this you need to train your body for two things. Correct breathing pattern and activating the right musculature of the core.

Breathing

The physiologically correct way to breathe is by using your diaphragm. Observe how children breathe. Their bellies are soft, they do not core if they are sticking out or not. We lose this ability as growing up we strive so hard to be sexy and beautiful, we forget to be healthy. Everybody's default is flexed abs. In a perfect world you would relearn to breathe through your belly and it is totally possible. However, for training considerations, you need to learn how to do this at least consciously and on command.

To perform a proper and deep breath, you need to inhale almost till you cannot take any more air in. The during the first two-thirds of the inhale, only your belly and lower ribs should expand, without chest moving at all. Only in the last one-third it is acceptable and desirable for your chest to move. Remember that taking a deep breath before performing a lift does not mean keeping air in your mouth. Let it out, as it may lead to problems after prolonged usage.

If you just can't perform a proper breathing pattern, try this progression. To get a sense of how it should feel, lie on your back and breathe deeply to the best of your abilities. You should notice that your belly moves considerably in this position. Try to remember the sensation and replicate it while sitting and then while standing. To open up the front of your body you may try some stretches. From simple lying on your back on a swissball with your arms above your head and then just try to breathe deeply, holding the air in for couple of seconds to allow a stretch.

Activating your abdominal wall

The simplest trick I can provide to make sure that you activate your muscles properly during different exercises is simply to constantly get reminded what to do. Let me explain – every time you do any movements that will activate you core (which is basically anything done not-lying down, as everything in real life outside of the gym) you should take a deep diaphragmatic breath and fill your belly with air (actually it's your organs coming down and full lungs push on them) pull your bellybutton towards your spine without flexing your abs. This will ensure that you've activated your transversus abdominis properly without unnecessary activation of the rectus abdominis. During heavy loading you will lose that ability and activate your six-pack muscles, however the more you can lift without it, the more functional your abdominal wall is and the less likely you are to suffer any problems.

As for the trick itself. I've seen some top-notch coaches do it, not only with regular Joes experiencing back pain but also with well-conditioned athletes. While you have your belly sucked in, wrap a piece of string around your waist. As soon as you will lose the activation, your belly will come out and push into the string. This will be a constant reminder to be tight and remain in control. During exercises like the squat, deadlift, overhead press, any standing pulling movement you should be able to perform without rectus abdominis activating up to a certain point. If you can't do even bodyweight squats without it jumping in, you really need to recondition your abdominal wall to work properly.

Chapter 11

Critical Stretches to Achieve Muscle Balance

Exercises themselves may not be enough to bring your body to proper balance. To facilitate the process, one should not only strengthen the weak muscles, but also stretch the shortened, tonic muscles to develop a well-rounded body. To achieve to goal of this book, it isn't needed to tie yourself in knots nor to do any elaborate stretching program. For 99% of people reading, a couple of simple stretches will be just enough. Remember – the objective is to have your iliac spines leveled and your head upright, with your ear just over your shoulder.

Neck extensors stretch

To stretch your neck extensors to reduce the forward head posture do the following. Stand tall with proper posture, clasp your hands behind your head and gently pull it towards your chest. To produce the fastest results, breathe deeply for 5 to 10 seconds and then try to pull your head up with your hands preventing it – your neck muscles should flex, but to motion should take place. After 5 seconds of flexing and holding your breath, exhale and release the tension. You should notice that you can pull your head further down. Repeat this protocol 3-5 times.

Upper abdominals stretch

Lie prone on the ground. Place your hand on the floor no farther than an inch or two from your chest, at the height of your solar plexus. Extend your arms pushing your trunk away from the floor, while keeping the pelvis firmly on the ground. Go only as far as you can without any great degree of discomfort, however far enough to feel the stretch. If you feel any pain, especially in your low back, take your time and progress very slowly. I remember that I couldn't do it due to pain at first, but as I progressed it became less of a nuisance and now I don't experience any discomfort whatsoever. Stay in the position for at least a minute, breathing deeply.

Hip flexor stretch

Stretch your hip flexors by kneeling on knee and then pushing your pelvis forward and down. Move your front foot so that your shin remains vertical. To be able to chill out more and allow the muscles to relax and lengthen, you may want to bend your torso down and place your hands on the floor. To control the whole position and not lose your balance, place books or blocks under your hands if needed. Rest in that position for at least a minute. If you feel too much of a discomfort to take it, you are probably overdoing it. Remember, stretching is seducing the muscles to go to sleep, not shouting to fall flat on their faces like a drill sergeant would.

Konrad Obidoski

Chapter 12
Progressive Core Exercises

In this chapter we're going to go over different exercises lined up in a difficulty sequence. If you cannot perform the previous level of intensity with adequate form, you should not move on to the next one. Each and every one of them should be performed while maintaining your intra-abdominal pressure and bellybutton brought towards your spine unless stated otherwise.

When creating a simple program for yourself always remember to structure it so that you train your lower abs first, then your obliques and your upper abs last. This way you will ensure proper recruitment and strengthening the weakest parts the most.

Lower abdominal exercises

Lower abdominal #1 – Finger pressure breathing

Lie back on the floor and put your hand palm-down under your back at the height of your bellybutton so that your spine presses slightly on your fingers. Tuck your butt under, so that your back flattens slightly. Bend your legs and place your feet on the ground. Gently pull your bellybutton towards your spine to activate the transverse muscles of the abdomen. Try not to flex anything else and as relaxed as you can inhale and hold this position for about 10 seconds for one rep. Your spine should press on your fingers the whole time, just hard enough to feel it. You goal is to make the pressure be constant and even.

Lower abdominal #2 – Finger pressure leg lowering

Lie back on the floor and put your hand palm-down under your back at the height of your bellybutton so that your spine presses slightly on your fingers. Tuck your butt under, so that your back flattens slightly. Bend your legs and place your feet on the ground. While keeping constant and gentle pressure on your fingers, raise one of your legs up to the point where your thigh is vertical. This is the starting position. To perform the exercise lower your leg until your lower back starts to arch. This is the end point of your movement. Obviously the more extended your leg is, the harder the exercise will become. Even more advanced version will have you put both of your legs up for starters and next lower them both at the same time. Insanely strong lower abs will allow your perform this exercise correctly even with weights between your ankles.

Lower abdominal #3 – Flat back knee raise

Lie back on the floor and tuck your butt under. Flex your hips so that your thighs are vertical and there is a 90 degree angle between your thighs and shins. While pulling your bellybutton towards your spine and maintaining a flat back try to lift your knees up. Even one centimeter movement is good. If you are doing this with perfect form, I can assure you that this won't be easy!

Lower abdominal #4 – Reverse crunch

To perform the reverse crunch you need to find a sturdy object you can hold on to with your hands. Have it above your head as you lie down on your back. Preferably do this exercise on a swissball or other curved surface that will allow full extension. Lie back on your ball fully extended and bring your thighs up so they create a 90 degree angle with your pelvis. Your knee joints should be maximally bent. Bring your knees towards your face by flexing the trunk and stop then your abdominal muscles are fully contracted. Do this exercise in a slow and controlled fashion.

Oblique exercises

Oblique #1 – Cable wood chop

Very popular exercise for athletes. Standing tall, grab the cable handle over your right shoulder with your right hand and with your left hand on top of it. Draw your bellybutton in and by rotating your torso and pulling with your arms bring the handle down to the height of your hips on the other side of your body. Obviously, as this is a bilateral exercise, you'll need to repeat for the other side. First I'd recommend learning this movement seated on a sturdy bench. Then standing up with your pelvis and legs fixed and finally while using more of a leg drive and shifting the weight of your body from one leg to the other to make it more of an integrated, full-body exercise.

Oblique #2 – Washing machine

Assume a wide and stable stance with your knees slightly bent. Grab a fairly light weight, bring it to your chest and hold on to it like to a child. Draw your bellybutton in and start rotating left and right far enough to stretch your obliques a little. At first do it slowly and then increase speed. You should stop the exercise when you are unable to maintain the speed you've built up to.

Oblique #3 – Russian twist

The only oblique exercise that most people I work with know of. Lie back on the floor and spread your arms to be stay stable. Your back should be flat on the ground. Start with your thighs vertical and your shins parallel to the floor. With your bellybutton drawn in, rotate your torso until you feel your shoulder lifting up. Don't let that happen. Harder variation of the exercise would be with your legs straight. You may also choose to use a swissball. To perform this version lie with your back on the ball and your feet on the floor with thighs parallel to the floor and a 90 degree angle in your knees. Clasp your hand together in front of you, with straight arms. You may choose to hold on to a weight if you're advanced. While keeping your butt tucked under and bellybutton drawn in, rotate left and right in a 180 degree spread.

Oblique #4 – Dumbbell side flexion

Stand tall with a dumbbell in one of your hands. While keeping your pelvis straight and bellybutton drawn in, bend sideways in the direction of the dumbbell and then in the opposite one, as far as you can, for full contraction. Keep your neck extended the whole time.

Oblique #5 – Ball side flexion

Lie on a swissball on your side. Put your feet wide to become stable. Your upper leg foot back and lower leg foot in front of you. Arms should be crossed on your chest. As you become more advanced, you can hold on to a weight plate. Extend fully on the ball and then curl up for full flexion of your obliques. You should have your torso in the frontal plane the whole time. Rotation is a sign of imbalance. Example: if your lie on your left side and right shoulder goes back during flexing up, it means that you have a tendency to rotate to your right. You can address that by doing more exercises that strengthen your left side rotation pattern. Remember, balance is key to enhancing performance and relieving pain.

Upper abdominal exercises

Upper abdominals #1 - Ball crunch

Lie back on the ball, with your head resting on it too, in full extension. Your shins should be vertical, with 90 degree angle in your knee joint. While maintaining a proper physiological position of the tongue and drawing your bellybutton in, flex forward until you reach full contraction of your abs. The easiest version is to have your arms in front of you, then to cross them on your chest and finally to place them on the sides of your head, with your fingers on the backs of your ears. They are not there to support your head!

Upper abdominals #2 – Cable crunch

Sit with on your heels with your back to the cable station. Use a rope instead of a handle and put each end of the rope on each of your shoulders. Grab them with your hands and have your forearms firmly pressed to your chest. Start with your torso at 45 degree angle to the floor. While crunching, your pelvis should remain stable, otherwise you are most likely using your hip flexors. To give yourself cues whether it is moving or not, you can place a swissball between your low back and the cable machine column.

Low back exercises

Low back #1 – Low back extensions

Lie on the back extension station and maintain straight back. While drawing your bellybutton in and extending your head, bend down and then slowly lift your trunk up. If you want to isolate the low back, keep your iliac spines on the bench so it stabilizes the pelvis. To make more of a whole extensor-chain exercise, move slightly up, to have your thighs on the bench. That will cause the force to be generated also with glutes and hamstrings. You can hold on to a weight with your arms if you want to make it more of a challenge. To provide even resistance throughout the whole movement, bring the weight to your chest at the top of the movement and get it over your head by straightening your arms while in the bottom portion. By manipulating the length of the lever arm, we achieve even force.

Low back #2 – Reverse hyperextensions

This exercise will provide more strain for the glutes, while reducing the load put on the low back. On the low back extension machine, lie with your stomach and your legs in the air, holding on to the pad with your hands. While keeping a neutral spine, start with your legs vertical. Lift one or both of your legs until the thighs are horizontal. Using both legs simultaneously as well as straightening them or adding weight will make the exercise more and more challenging.

Sample exercise program

Basically every abs exercise program can be structured similarly to this template. Say you train at gym 3 times a week, on Monday, Wednesday and Friday. After each session you can perform an abs workout. Example:

Monday – 1-2 sets of 2 exercises for lower abs and obliques and 1-2 sets of one exercise for upper abs. Wednesday – 2 sets of 2 exercises for lower abs and obliques and 2 sets of one exercise for upper abs. Friday – 2 sets of 2 exercises for lower abs and obliques and 2 sets of one exercise for upper abs.

Or:

Monday – 2-3 sets of 2 exercises for lower abs or 1-2 sets of 3 exercises for lower abs. Wednesday – 2-3 sets of 2 exercises for obliques or 1-2 sets of 3 exercises for obliques.

Friday – 2-3 sets of 2 exercises for upper abs or 1-2 sets of 3 exercises for upper abs.

If your problem is a flat back instead of the most common overarched one, you can replace the low abs with low back exercises to fix it. Play with it and see what gives you best results. Be smart and do not overdo it.

Konrad Obidoski

Conclusion

Thank you again for Purchasing this book!

If used correctly this book may help you with all your athletic endeavors as core is the basis for all strength generation. If you are not an athlete, it should help you greatly in reducing any pains you may experience that will diminish your quality of life.

The next step is to create a program for yourself or use the sample one if applicable and simply start exercising and begin that step-by-step progression.

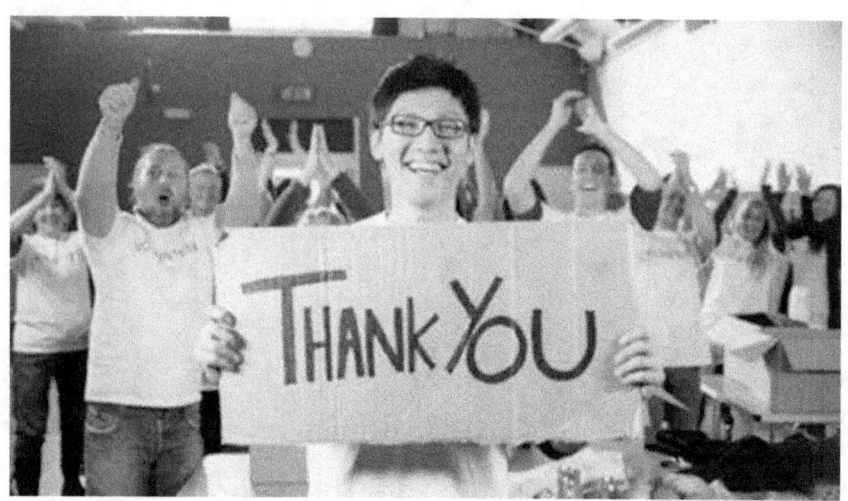

If you enjoyed this book, then I'd like to ask you for a favor that won't cost you anything and help me a tremendous amount. Would you be kind enough to leave a review for this book on Amazon? It'd be greatly appreciated!

Preview of "Bodyweight Training: Best Bodyweight Exercises to Build Muscle and Lose Fat Fast"

Introduction

First of all, I want to thank you and congratulate you for Purchasing the book, "Bodyweight Training: Best Bodyweight Exercises To Build Muscle And Lose Fat Fast".

This book contains a proven strategy on how to utilize bodyweight training to its full extent and achieve an impressive physique without the necessity of using any equipment.

Let's get something straight. Training is training, resistance is resistance, whether you use the weight of your body or the weight of a barbell – it does not matter. If you follow basic principles of effective training you will get the results. The problem is that most people do not understand them or fail to apply them to bodyweight training. After all a push-up is a push-up, you can't change the intensity of it, you can just do more and more of them, right? Dead wrong! There are many variations that will allow you to do just that. Without progressive overload your physique and strength gains will be seriously compromised.

This book will teach you how to use basic training principles that decide whether you will be adding muscle to your bones and loosing fat. You will learn how to utilize training variables and manipulate them to achieve the outcome you are aiming for. You will be armed to the teeth with enough knowledge to enjoy any kind of physique you want.

Thanks again for Purchasing this book, I hope you enjoy it and I know it will bring you results if you only apply the information and work hard enough!

Let's do this!

Chapter 1: Setting your training objectives

Ever heard the phrase "you can't hit a target you cannot see"? Before you apply anything you need to know the optimal strategy and before you work it out, you need to know what you want to achieve.

This book is primarily focusing on hypertrophy or building muscle and loosing that unnecessary fat. However you can use the contents to pursue other athletic goals. To determine them it is best to go through a simple 5–step thought process:

1. Think of the one thing that causes you most pain in your physique or your athletic ability. Do you feel weak? Overweight? Skinny? Whatever it is, know your weaknesses and then employ a strategy that will allow you to fight and win again it!

2. If you know what thing you need to overcome to increase the quality of your life the most, set up a positive statement that will inspire and encourage you to pursue it. Don't say "I am weak" or "I am fat". Say "I am STRONG!", "I am a sexy devil!". This will create a mindset you will need to stick with it! Preferably repeat it as frequently as possible!

3. Establish a concrete goals. Use a well-known SMART formula. The goal must be Specific, Measurable,

Attainable, Realistic and Time-constrained. If you are a beginner, you may for example have such goal: "I will perform one pull-up at the end of the month". It's not too big to terrify you, you can clearly see when it is achieved and by when you want it to be achieved.

4. Chunk them down as needed. If you have a goal to perform 100 push-ups but a of now you can do only 10, have a goal each month to increase that number by 5, 10, whatever you think is realistic and attainable.

5. Go after them and stay at it! Even if you miss a deadline, even if you encounter more roadblocks that expected – KEEP. AT. IT. Nothing ever was accomplished by people who quit at the first sign of trouble. Don't be one of these people.

Warning!

This book is meant for educational purposes only and any responsibility of using included contents lies upon the reader. Every physical activity carries a potential risk of injury and therefore it is best to consult a physician before starting any exercise program to ensure a sufficient level of health and fitness to continue. No liability is assumed for the information contained herein.

Konrad Obidoski

www.ingramcontent.com/pod-product-compliance
Lightning Source LLC
Chambersburg PA
CBHW062010280526
45787CB00005B/2049